Healthy *and* Beautiful *with* COCONUT OIL

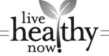

Cynthia Holzapfel
Laura Holzapfel

HEALTHY LIVING PUBLICATIONS
Summertown, Tennessee

© 2014 Cynthia Holzapfel, Laura Holzapfel

Cover and interior design: Scattaregia Design

Healthy Living Publications,
a division of Book Publishing Company
P.O. Box 99
Summertown, TN 38483
888-260-8458
bookpubco.com

ISBN: 978-1-57067-314-6

Printed in the United States of America

19 18 17 16 15 14   1 2 3 4 5 6 7 8 9

Library of Congress Cataloging-in-Publication Data

Holzapfel, Cynthia, 1948-
 Healthy and beautiful with coconut oil / Cynthia Holzapfel, Laura Holzapfel.
    pages cm
 Includes bibliographical references.
 ISBN 978-1-57067-314-6 (pbk.) -- ISBN 978-1-57067-883-7 (e-book)
 1. Coconut oil--Health aspects--Popular works. 2. Fatty acids in human nutrition. 3. Coconut oil--Therapeutic use. I. Holzapfel, Laura. II. Title.
 QP144.O44H66 2014
 612.3'97--dc23
                        2014024334

Printed on recycled paper

Book Publishing Company is a member of Green Press Initiative. We chose to print this title on paper with 100% post consumer recycled content, processed without chlorine, which saved the following natural resources:

• 18 trees

• 563 pounds of solid waste

• 8,414 gallons of water

• 1,551 pounds of greenhouse gases

• 8 million BTU of energy

For more information on Green Press Initiative, visit www.greenpressinitiative.org. Environmental impact estimates were made using the Environmental Defense Fund Paper Calculator. For more information visit www.papercalculator.org.

CONTENTS

The Interest in Coconut Oil

Coconut oil has been used in food preparation for many years, and with good reason. Coconut oil is a stable saturated fat, which means it keeps baked goods fresh and doesn't break down when used to fry foods. Half a century ago, when saturated fat was implicated as a possible cause for heart disease, all the saturated tropical oils, including coconut oil, palm kernel oil, and palm oil, earned the same unfavorable reputation as saturated animal fats. The consequence of this negative publicity was a sharp decline in the use of coconut oil in commercial foods and consumer resistance to using it at home. Proponents of coconut oil also cite the growing concern of the American vegetable oil industry, primarily the processors of soy oil, about competition from coconut oil. Industry pressure may have exerted influence on public policy and scientific research to discredit its use.

We believe coconut oil has many benefits, and we hope this book will clarify why we feel its revival is justified. Coconut oil is getting more attention from researchers because of its proven ability to reduce bacterial and viral infection, so we'll review the results of some of this research. In addition, we'll provide some delicious recipes that incorporate coconut oil and explain how to use coconut products in beauty formulas.

A Comparison of Fats

There's a lot of conflicting information about which fats and oils are the best for health. Should you only use olive oil or canola oil? Is margarine good for your heart or not? Are animal fats all that bad and do they actually contribute to a well-balanced diet? The answers are easier to understand if you know a little about what goes into the composition of different fats and how your body processes them.

A Bit of Fat Chemistry

All fats are made up of combinations of carbon and hydrogen atoms. The qualities of each fat are determined by how many carbon and hydrogen atoms the fat molecule has and how these atoms are arranged. If the arrangement is chemically stable, the fat is called saturated. A saturated fat is usually solid at room temperature and is less susceptible to chemical reactions that would alter its makeup. Examples of fats containing a lot of saturates are butter, lard, and other animal fats; peanut oil; and coconut oil.

If the chemical composition of a fat is not as stable as a saturated fat, it's called unsaturated. Unsaturated fats are usually liquid at room temperature and can have either one point of instability (monounsaturated) or several points (polyunsaturated). Olive oil contains a high amount of monounsaturates. Common polyunsaturated oils are corn, flaxseed, safflower, soy, and sunflower, as well as oils from fish.

You may hear certain oils referred to as "saturated" or "polyunsaturated" and get the impression that those oils are completely one type or another. In reality, most fats and oils are made up of a combination of saturates and unsaturates, including different types of each of those. Although animal fats and tropical oils, such as coconut oil, are very high in saturates and most vegetable oils are high in unsaturates, even beef fat is composed of almost half unsaturates and corn oil contains almost 15 percent saturated fat.

It's important to note that the saturated fat in coconut oil has a different chemical composition than saturates in meat and dairy products. Researchers believe this unique composition sets coconut oil apart from other saturated fats and contributes to its healing properties.

Chemically Altered Fats

In the early 1900s, chemists were looking for a cheap alternative to butter and shortening. Modern oil-processing techniques made liquid oils plentiful and inexpensive. Scientists discovered that liquid oils could be converted into a solid form if the structure of carbon and hydrogen molecules in those oils was changed. As a result, the desirable characteristics of a saturated fat could be created, even though the fat would still be fundamentally unsaturated. Two common types of artificial solid fats are trans fats and hydrogenated fats.

Trans Fats

For the most part, trans fats are processed from polyunsaturated fats to have properties that more closely resemble saturated fats. Trans fats were created in order to replace either saturated fats that were in short supply, such as butter during war times, or unstable polyunsaturated fats in baked goods to prolong their freshness on supermarket shelves.

There are a few naturally occurring trans fats in some animal fats, but most trans fats are created from polyunsaturates by chemically altering them with heat and pressure. Molecules of trans fats have the same straight, rigid structure that molecules of saturated fats have, and this structure is what makes both fats solid at room temperature. An inexpensive solid fat is a boon to food manufacturers, as they can use it not only to make processed foods more cheaply but to also extend their shelf lives.

There's a twist, however—both literally and figuratively. Although a trans fat has the chemical composition of an unsaturated fat, the altered structure of the artificial molecule is twisted, so that the atoms aren't aligned the same way they are in the unsaturated fat. This unnatural structure makes it difficult for our bodies to assimilate trans fats. The sensitive human biochemical system treats trans fats the way it would unsaturated fats, but the altered structure of trans fats prevents proper metabolism. Trans fats take up the space normally reserved for unaltered unsaturated fats and block certain processes from occurring. This disruption can cause problems with heartbeat regulation, cell division, neuron firing, mental stability, sense functions, and overall well-being.

Hydrogenated Fats

Hydrogenation is another artificial process used to transform liquid oils into solid fats. During this process, heat, pressure, and hydrogen gas are used to add extra hydrogen atoms to the chains of carbon atoms, creating a rigid, stable fat. Partial hydrogenation occurs when only part of the fat molecule is filled with extra hydrogen. By filling only part of a molecule, chemists can control the solidity of the artificial fat; the more hydrogen added, the more solid the fat will be.

The process of hydrogenation disrupts the original chemical composition of unsaturated fats, resulting in altered substances that are harmful to our bodies. It's impossible to completely control the chemical reactions that occur during hydrogenation or ensure that only a minimal amount of these unwanted molecules is produced. Trans fats also are created during hydrogenation.

The Case for Avoiding Chemically Altered Fats

Foods processed with chemically altered trans fats and hydrogenated fats have become very popular. Manufacturers love these fats because products made with them are less prone to spoilage. Food processors can also more closely control how these foods look and taste. In some cases, altered fats are much less expensive than the solid fats they replace. Even though coconut oil could fill much of this niche without having to be processed, the large supply of vegetable oils in the United States has encouraged growth in the production of artificially solid vegetable fats. Unfortunately, this financial savings for manufacturers comes at great cost to our health.

The Role of Fats

Our principal source of energy comes from the fats in our diets. These fats contain about 9 calories per gram; carbohydrates and protein contain only 4 calories per gram. Simply put, protein builds tissues and carbohydrates provide an immediate source of energy for physical exertion and are essential for brain function. Accumulated fats in the body provide a storage repository of energy when carbohydrate intake isn't adequate. In extreme situations, these fat stores protect us from starvation. It may be hard to imagine needing this type of survival mechanism in modern times of plenty, when so many of us are tempted by high-calorie treats. However, the ability to store fat was absolutely essential for our ancestors, whose food supplies were not always dependable or nutritious. It's so important for the body to have a supply of fat to draw on, that even during times of starvation, it will try to retain a certain amount of fat.

Fats help diminish feelings of hunger. They're digested more slowly than protein or carbohydrates and are a concentrated source of calories that helps regulate the body's "appestat," or appetite thermometer. In the ancient diets of our ancestors, before processed, refined ingredients were invented, the consumption of a certain amount of fats triggered a signal that meant "enough calories for now, thank you."

By surrounding vital organs and cushioning bones, fat also provides protection from the jostling caused by daily activities and the shock of impact when we walk, sit, and handle hard objects. An adequate layer of fat under the skin also protects us from the cold.

Fats literally shape who we are, because they play a role in forming secondary sex characteristics. Men tend to put on more abdominal fat than women, and women have larger deposits of subcutaneous fat (the fat that lies directly beneath the skin), as well as fat in the buttocks, thighs, and breasts. A prevalent belief is that the particular distribution of fat in a woman's body is related to her biological role in childbearing. In other words, enough fat ensures that she'll have an adequate supply of fat in her breast milk and plenty of calories for growing a baby.

Metabolizing Fats

Most fats are metabolized, or broken down, in the liver. From there, smaller fat molecules, as well as cholesterol, are carried through the bloodstream by one of two substances: high-density lipoproteins or low-density lipoproteins. "Density" refers to the amount of protein in these molecules; a lipoprotein is a combination of protein and fat. You may be more familiar with the abbreviations of these terms: HDL and LDL. LDL transports cholesterol to artery walls to repair damage; HDL removes cholesterol from artery walls and returns it to the liver so it can be eliminated from the body if it's not needed. You'll often see HDL and LDL referred to as "cholesterol," but this is shorthand for "cholesterol carried by high-density or low-density lipoproteins."

Fats that aren't metabolized shortly after digestion are stored in fat cells under the skin (adipose tissue), as is any excess carbohydrate. A certain amount of carbohydrate can be stored in muscle cells and in the liver for quick use, but once the liver has taken in all it can hold, it converts this carbohydrate into stored fat.

Not all fats take the same route through the digestive process. Fats made up of small molecules, known as short-chain fatty acids (those with fewer than eight carbons) and medium-chain fatty acids (those with eight to fourteen carbons), are absorbed directly into the blood and transported to the liver. Most, but not all, of these short- and medium-chain fatty acids are saturated fats from both animal and plant sources. They're used quickly and primarily as a source of energy, as opposed to longer saturated and unsaturated fat molecules. As a result, people with liver problems find short-chain saturated fatty acids easier to digest, because those molecules require less work by the liver to break up and recombine for use in the body.

Long-chain fatty acids (those with twelve or more carbons) are converted into smaller fats in the intestine and take more work to break down so they can be absorbed in the bloodstream. Most, but not all, of these long-chain fatty acids are unsaturated fats. These fats have a special role: keeping the cell membranes fluid. They also create an environment that's inhospitable to bacteria and viruses and help move electrical impulses in the body.

The longer saturated-fat molecules have a greater tendency to aggregate, or cluster, and hold together. Their positive role in the body is to help form the structure of cell membranes. On the downside, they also form plaques, the sticky substances that gather around injured areas in artery walls and contribute to clogged arteries.

The Role of Cholesterol

Although cholesterol isn't a fat, it's so often mentioned along with discussions of fat that many people think they are one and the same. Cholesterol is actually a waxy substance created in the body from small molecules that form after fats and sugars are broken down. We also can get cholesterol from eating animal products; it's never found in plant foods. Healthy individuals usually produce all the cholesterol they need. However, there's evidence that some people, such as the elderly, can't make enough cholesterol and may benefit from the addition of some cholesterol in their diets.

Cholesterol has gotten a bad reputation over the years because of its association with heart disease. But like many natural substances, cholesterol isn't all bad. It's essential for helping cell membranes retain their structure. Cholesterol is also a building block for vitamin D and certain hormones, especially the hormones that regulate sexual functioning: estrogen, progesterone, and testosterone. In addition, cholesterol is used to make stress hormones. When the body is under stress, more cholesterol is created to form adrenal hormones that prepare us to either fight or flee the source of stress.

There's definitely evidence that high levels of cholesterol in the blood are associated with the hardened arteries and arterial blockages that lead to heart disease, but there's disagreement among experts as to whether eating foods high in cholesterol causes this condition. It would seem to make sense that people could lower the amount of cholesterol in their blood by consuming less cholesterol in the foods they eat. But study after study has been unable to demonstrate a significant correspondence between cholesterol consumption and blood cholesterol levels.

Some researchers have focused on trans fats as a cause of high cholesterol levels, theorizing that the presence of these fats crowds out natural fats that would help the body maintain normal, healthful amounts of cholesterol. Other experts are looking at whether an overabundance of free radicals (unstable molecules that are created during normal biological processes) can create artery damage that's repaired by cholesterol. An accumulation of cholesterol at any one site of damage could cause blockage in that blood vessel. A lack of certain vitamins and other antioxidants may lead to higher levels of free radicals and in turn create conditions that would lead to the production of more serum cholesterol.

Looking beyond cholesterol as a cause of heart disease, some experts have pointed to high levels of omega-6 fatty acids, which are found in corn, cottonseed, safflower, soybean, and sunflower oils. Oils rich in omega-6 fatty acids have been promoted widely over the last thirty years as healthful alternatives to saturated fats, but we now know that these fats can cause increased blood pressure, inflammation, and blood clots.

The Relationship Between Saturated Fats and Cholesterol Levels

For many years it was thought that saturated fat increased cholesterol levels. When measurements of cholesterol levels in the blood were first done, only the total of both helpful HDL and harmful LDL were recorded. It was assumed that the presence of both indicated high levels of cholesterol. Now that testing has become more sophisticated, researchers take into account the balance of these two types and note whether a food or medication raises cholesterol only when HDL levels are low or when LDL levels are high. In some cases, certain foods lower total cholesterol levels, but they tend to do so only by lowering HDL quite a bit while simultaneously raising levels of LDL.

For a long time, saturated fat was also thought to increase the incidence of heart disease, but the data collected from several significant studies on saturates and coronary disease don't confirm a direct correlation. As a result, some cardiovascular researchers are questioning this long-held belief. Prominent in this group of researchers is Walter Willett, MD, DrPH, of Harvard University, himself a longtime proponent of the relationship between saturated fat and heart disease. Willet participated in a study of over 43,000 health professionals who had no prior incidence of heart disease or diabetes. The study concluded the following:

Diets high in saturated fat and cholesterol are associated with an increased risk of coronary disease, but these adverse effects are at least in part explained by their low fiber content and association with other risk factors. Benefits of reducing intakes of saturated fat and cholesterol are likely to be modest unless accompanied by an increased consumption of foods rich in fiber.[1]

Although saturated fats, especially the saturated fats in animal products, tend to clump together in the arteries, eating saturated fats may not in and of itself increase the risk of blocked arteries, heart disease, and stroke. However, eating a lot of vegetable oil high in omega-6 fatty acids can increase the risk of conditions that often lead to heart disease, including high blood pressure, inflammation, blood clotting, and even cancer (cell proliferation). Eating a diet that's high in essential omega-3 fatty acids from whole-food sources, such as flaxseeds, hempseeds, walnuts, and even dark leafy greens, provides a good balance for diets that include saturated fats and other polyunsaturated vegetable oils.

In summary, heart disease may result from a number of causes, and what produces heart disease in one person may not affect another person in the same way. A study at the Cleveland Clinic that examined 120,000 heart patients concluded that diabetes, high blood pressure, high cholesterol, and smoking are the most important overall risk factors for heart disease. Based on current research, the best advice is to eat a diet high in natural, unprocessed foods and not participate in behaviors that could elevate health risks.

Nutritive Benefits of Coconut Oil

Coconut oil has many good qualities in its favor. Because it's a naturally solid, saturated fat that doesn't easily become rancid at room temperature or break down with high heat, it can be used to enhance baked goods and fry foods. Besides being a valuable ingredient in food preparation, coconut oil has specific health benefits that make it worthwhile to add to your diet.

Coconut oil makes an excellent replacement for trans fats in processed foods. Over the years, trans fats have been implicated in a growing array of health problems, primarily heart disease. A number of studies have shown that trans fats increase LDL and decrease HDL. In a study published in the Netherlands, researchers looked at the effects of replacing animal fats and hydrogenated oils with palm oil, another saturated tropical oil similar to coconut oil.[2] Although the diet using palm oil didn't lower total cholesterol levels, it did lower LDL cholesterol by 8 percent and increased HDL cholesterol by 11 percent, bringing the balance of the two toward more healthy levels. A more recent study also done in the Netherlands showed that replacing foods containing trans fats with those containing saturated fats (particularly foods in which lauric acid, the primary fat in coconut oil, made up about one-third of the saturates) also improved HDL cholesterol levels.[3]

Inflammation, Digestion, and Other Health Problems

Coconut oil may be helpful in reducing inflammation, the body's response to infection. A British study tested the response of mice to a five-week diet that was either low in fat or high in one of the following oils: coconut, olive, safflower, or fish oil. The mice on all the diets were exposed to pathogens. The results showed that both coconut oil and fish oil did more to diminish inflammation in the mice than any of the other fats they were fed, leading the researchers to believe that "both these fatty acids might be useful thera-pies in acute and chronic inflammatory diseases."[4]

Because the medium-chain fatty acids found in coconut oil are more quickly digested than long-chain saturated fatty acids, they're often a good choice for individuals who have digestive disorders or more delicate digestive systems, such as infants or the elderly. Mother's milk has a high content of lauric acid (a medium-chain fatty acid); consequently, nutrition-ists are considering coconut oil a good food for babies because it also has a high proportion of lauric acid. A number of studies have been conducted on the healthful properties of adding coconut oil to infant formula. In one such study done at the University of Iowa, researchers compared how well fat and calcium were absorbed by infants.[5] The infant formulas they used contained either palm oil (which is predominantly composed of palmitic and oleic acids, both unsaturated fats) or coconut oil. They found a signifi-cant improvement in absorption when the babies were fed formula rich in coconut oil.

Coconut oil may also be beneficial for people who suffer from Crohn's disease, a disorder marked by inflammation of the intestines, and people with ulcerative colitis, a similar disease affecting the colon. Research has been done showing that the anti-inflammatory properties of coconut oil are effective at reducing the irritation created by Crohn's disease. In addi-tion, coconut oil's antimicrobial properties (which are explored more in the next section) may be effective in fighting the bacteria and viruses often cited as a cause of Crohn's disease, stomach ulcers, and other ulcerative diseases of the intestinal tract. People who struggle with digestive diseases find it easy to assimilate coconut oil, making it easier for them to eat nutri-tious foods and regain their health.[6]

Another potential use for coconut oil may be the treatment of benign (noncancerous) enlarged prostate in men. A currently popular and successful herbal treatment for this condition includes the use of saw palmetto berries. These berries contain a substance that inhibits dihydrotestosterone (DHT), which is derived from testosterone and increases in men as they age. DHT is thought to be responsible for cell growth in the prostate, leading to its enlargement. The active ingredient in saw palmetto berries is believed to contain medium-chain fatty acids that might help block the conversion of testosterone to DHT. It's possible that coconut oil, with its high content of medium-chain fatty acids, may also have a positive effect on prostatitis and enlarged prostate.[7]

High Metabolism and Weight Loss

Coconut oil may contribute to weight loss in several ways. An excellent report was published in the *Journal of Nutrition* on whether medium-chain fatty acids could be used to prevent obesity.[8] The authors presented an overview of almost thirty studies on the various effects of medium-chain fatty acids on metabolism, satiety (the sensation of fullness after eating), body fat, and body weight. Most, but not all, of the studies in their compilation showed an increase in metabolism when subjects followed diets high in medium-chain fatty acids in which 30 to 40 percent of the calories came from fat. The effects of medium-chain fatty acids on satiety were somewhat less clear, but the studies still indicated that medium-chain fatty acids might decrease appetite.

There's also a possibility that eating coconut oil can reduce white fatty tissue, the layer of fat below the skin that so often accumulates around the waistline (as opposed to the brown fatty adipose tissue that surrounds internal organs). In a study conducted in Spain, researchers varied the fat and calorie content of diets fed to rats, enriching one of the test diets with coconut oil. Their results showed that the diet high in coconut oil stimulated a cell component called uncoupling protein (UCP1), essential for the processing of food into energy in cells. In this way, coconut oil actually helped to reduce subcutaneous fat stores in the rats in this study.[9]

Saturated Coconut Oil as a Safe Food

Few people had any opinions about the healthfulness of coconut oil until a negative assessment of it by the Center for Science in the Public Interest (CSPI) was widely publicized in the early 1990s. The focus of this publicity was the use of coconut oil on movie theater popcorn, as well as its addition to baked goods. CSPI has conducted many informative campaigns, such as exposing nutritional deficiencies in the processed foods available in supermarkets and the high calorie content of restaurant dishes. However, this is one instance where the watchdog organization may have jumped on the bandwagon against saturated fat before doing its homework. At the very least, a consideration of the health of large groups of people who have made coconut oil their principal fat source for generations would have led to a very different conclusion about whether coconut oil should be demonized.

Proponents of coconut oil point out that many of the studies condemning the saturated fat in tropical oils have been done using refined tropical oils. This would eliminate some of the health-supporting properties found in the unrefined oil traditionally consumed by native populations in tropical areas. Coconut oil was also blamed for increasing cholesterol levels and heart disease in a number of animal experiments. But in these experiments, the animals also were on diets that restricted the amount of essential fats needed to help prevent the incidence of these health problems, so the results of the studies were probably more reflective of a lack of essential fats than of problems with coconut oil.[10]

A number of more positive studies have been carried out in India and Southeast Asia, where consumption of coconut oil is at some of the highest levels in the world. In southern India, fresh and dried coconut and coconut oil are staples in the diet. The traditional diet in India is much lower in fat than Western diets, but coronary artery disease is rising significantly, much in the same way that it is in regions of the world where diets are high in fat, especially saturated fat. P. D. Kumar, a researcher from the south Indian state of Kerala, compared a group of Indians with coronary artery disease with a control group of healthy individuals and discovered that the consumption of coconut oil in both groups was about the same.[11] The presence of coconut oil in the diet did not increase the risk for arteriosclerosis; in fact, when the amount of coconut meat in the diet was increased, harmful LDL cholesterol levels actually dropped.

In Malaysia, researchers looked at the effects of controlled diets containing proportionally high amounts of coconut oil, corn oil, or palm oil.[12] They found that while coconut oil raised the total amount of cholesterol in the blood, it did so by raising the ratio of good HDL cholesterol to harmful LDL cholesterol. Although both corn oil and palm oil reduced total cholesterol, they also reduced the proportion of HDL cholesterol—a factor that researchers feel is a more important risk factor for heart disease. Similar results were seen when the fats found in coconut oil—lauric acid and myristic acid—were increased in the diets of healthy men. Again, although total cholesterol increased slightly, the rise was due in large part to the increase of vital HDL levels, a positive factor for health.[13]

Agronomist P. K. Thampan has written extensively about the research studies that evaluate coconut oil consumption and health in Southeast Asia. He noted that in Sri Lanka alone, the average consumption of coconuts is about 90 per person annually (about one-quarter of one coconut every day)—and that's just for whole coconut. The amount increases to 120 coconuts each year per person when the amount of coconut oil consumed is taken into account, making Sri Lanka an excellent place to study coconut oil's effects. Thampan describes a study of sixteen young men who were fed a diet in which coconut oil and other coconut products were the main sources of fat. The same men were then fed a diet where the principal fats were from dairy products and corn oil. Measurements of the blood fat levels of the study's participants showed that the corn oil diet lowered total cholesterol levels but also lowered levels of good HDL cholesterol. However, the diet high in coconut fat not only kept total cholesterol at a healthy level (around 180), it kept HDL levels high relative to LDL levels.[14, 15]

Perhaps the most quoted study on this subject was carried out by Ian Prior on the Polynesian islands of Pukapuka and Tokelau, where coconut oil is a major source of fat in the diet. Coconut oil contributes 35 to 56 percent of calories compared to US recommendations of 30 percent of calories from all fat sources.[16] Because of this, the amount of saturated fat in the diet is quite high, but the incidence of cardiovascular disease is very low. Cholesterol levels ranged from 170 to 180 on Pukapuka to between 210 and 215 on Tokelau, where overall fat consumption was the greatest. Notably, heart disease was not a common health problem for the people on these islands, even with the large amount of saturated plant fat they consumed.

The Case Against Polyunsaturates

Eating a diet too high in polyunsaturates may be more harmful to health than eating the saturated fats in coconut oil. Several recent studies show that it may be unhealthy to consume oils extracted from nuts and seeds because these oils are lacking the protective nutrients that accompanied them in their whole, natural state. Nuts and seeds contain a number of compounds that fight cancer and heart disease. The fiber in nuts and seeds also helps reduce the incidence of diabetes, as long as total fat intake is moderate. Perhaps most important, though, is how the protective shells and skins on nuts and seeds minimize how quickly the oils they contain degrade or spoil. Once polyunsaturated oils are isolated from their whole-food sources, they tend to break down and become unstable. The result of this instability is the formation of free radicals, the harmful substances that can create cell damage in the body.

Coconut Oil in a Healthful Plant-Based Diet

Much of the research on the relationship between saturated fats and heart disease points to the possibility that saturated fats and cholesterol in animal products may play more of a role in causing health problems than saturated fats in plant foods. However, even as researchers uncover more information about the role of nutrition in health, it has become less clear why certain foods seem to cause or prevent disease. Heredity plays a key role in shaping our biology and determining to what degree we're susceptible to certain health problems. Although the consumption of cholesterol and saturated animal fat can lead to high cholesterol levels and heart disease, there are scores of people whose cholesterol levels are not adversely affected this way.

Many medical professionals believe that whether saturated fats and cholesterol adversely affect health depends on how these substances are consumed. Are they eaten as whole foods or as part of a diet rich in whole foods, or is the diet largely composed of refined foods? Even the Harvard University study quoted on page 13 indicates that eating whole plant foods might play a significant role in protecting individuals from heart disease, regardless of their consumption of foods high in cholesterol or saturated fat.

For many years, the nutritional recommendation for people with diabetes was to reduce the amount of sugar and other carbohydrates they consumed. In more recent years, diabetes research has become more sophisticated, and there's growing concern that the amount of fat people are eating is contributing to an increased incidence of diabetes. It's impossible to ignore the current epidemic of obesity and the fact that being overweight increases the risk of contracting diabetes, affirming that no singular food group is the culprit when it comes to this terrible disease. Researchers have measured the effects of a variety of foods on blood sugar levels and discovered that unprocessed, high-fiber foods do the best job of regulating blood sugar, no matter if these foods are primarily carbohydrates, fats, or protein. This revelation also makes a good case for eating a wide variety of whole plant foods in general, rather than focusing on one food group or one nutritional component as being either all good or all bad.

Does the inclusion of fresh coconut in the diet help boost the healthful properties of coconut oil? P. K. Thampan suggests that the benefits of coconut oil can be optimized by including it in a whole-food, plant-based diet:

All the edible components of coconut contribute substantially to the dietary calories of people in the major coconut growing and consuming countries. The edible components are also good sources of protein, fiber, and minerals. This could be the reason why people consuming large amounts of coconut and coconut oil in a varied diet in different parts of the world do not demonstrate hypercholesterolaemia [high cholesterol levels] and coronary heart disease.

The only limitation in the dietary use of coconut oil is its low content of essential fatty acids. This deficiency will not, however, become manifest when people consume a normal diet containing cereals, pulses [beans and other legumes], roots and tubers, fish, etc., which are good sources of these acids. Coconut oil and coconut kernel [coconut meat] as dietary components sustain optimum levels of vitamin E in people besides causing enhanced secretion of insulin and utilization of blood glucose.[17]

We support this conclusion and urge you try out the cookbooks listed on page 46, which feature whole-food dishes using coconut and coconut oil.

Antimicrobial Properties of Coconut Oil

In the past 150 years, there have been significant advancements in the fight against infectious diseases. Even with this progress, outbreaks still persist and previously unknown diseases continue to surface. One such instance occurred in 1993 in Milwaukee, Wisconsin, with the contamination of the municipal water supply. It resulted in an outbreak of cryptosporidiosis, a parasitic infection in the intestine that affected an estimated 400,000 people. Roughly 4,400 of those who were infected required hospitalization.[18]

Although scientists had predicted that the fight against infectious diseases would have been won by now, the arrival of new viruses and the reemergence of previously defeated illnesses continue to plague the medical community. In the 1992 Institute of Medicine report *Emerging Infections: Microbial Threats to Health in the United States*, it was noted that the death rate for infectious diseases rose 58 percent from 1980 to 1992.[19] Besides the ability of microbes to adapt and change, the reasons listed for this increase included the escalation of international travel for people, animals, and traded goods; changing land use patterns; human demographics; and the breakdown of public health infrastructures to deal with infectious disease problems.

The Problem of Antibiotic Resistance

A major factor in the increase of hospitalization and death rates from infectious diseases is the rise in antibiotic resistance in different types of bacteria. Many people expect to get an antibiotic each time they visit the doctor, as if it were the magic bullet for any ailment. Unfortunately, bacteria and other microscopic organisms can adapt so effectively that they can resist the drugs that are used to fight them. As a result, doctors have had to resort to using stronger and stronger antibiotics in order to cure infectious diseases.

Anytime you take an antibiotic, you increase the risk that harmful bacteria will become resistant to that particular medication. If you increase the potency of the antibiotics you take, you also increase the risk of harboring more-potent bacteria.

Some bacteria have the ability to share information with other organisms, including how to become resistant to different antibiotics. Even if the harmful bacteria inside us don't cause us to become ill, chances are increasing that they are resistant to antibiotics and could pass on this resistance to a different and extremely dangerous organism. For example, you might be harboring a relatively benign form of *E. coli* virus, but if that virus comes in contact with a drug-resistant organism, it could assimilate the information it needs to become a virulent form of *E. coli*, capable of causing a life-threatening illness that doesn't respond to antibiotics.

Antibiotic resistance has become endemic. The American Medical Association studied this sweeping trend and concluded that the global increase in resistance to antimicrobial drugs, including the resistance of emerging bacterial strains to all currently available antibacterial agents, is creating a public health problem that could potentially reach crisis proportions.

There is also considerable overuse of antibiotics in animal feed. For the past fifty years, farmers have fed cattle, pigs, and poultry low levels of antibiotics with the hope that this would reduce the infections caused by their cramped living quarters. In 1998, the European Union instituted recommendations proposed by the World Health Organization and banned the use of antibiotics as growth promoters in the food-animal industry. Note that these same antibiotics are commonly prescribed for the treatment of human infections.

Workers in the meat-packing industry regularly come in contact with resistant microbes as a result of handling animal carcasses in slaughterhouses and often develop illnesses that can only be cured with very strong antibiotics. When they become ill, packing plant workers have an increased chance of spreading these resistant germs to their families and friends. Meat-packing plants traditionally have had a poor record for maintaining safe, sanitary conditions, both for their workers and during the processing of the product itself, and meat is easily contaminated in these less-than-ideal conditions.

Eighty percent of illnesses caused by known pathogens are actually initiated by viruses. Vaccines have contributed immensely to the eradication of many viruses. But to be effective, a vaccine must be administered before a person gets sick, and only a select number of viruses have associated vaccines. Although there are antiviral drugs on the market, not one of them effectively destroys viruses; therefore, they are unable to cure the illnesses viruses cause. All that antiviral drugs do is slow the growth of the viral invasion; your natural defenses still need to fight off the infection.

Our intention is not to cause undue concern with this information. At one time or another, nearly all of us have been afflicted with bacterial or viral illnesses that were not life-threatening. If your immune system is working properly, you should be able to fight off these illnesses with little, if any, use of antibiotics. But the growing overuse of antibiotics, and the subsequent rise of antibiotic resistance, should encourage you to investigate other ways to protect and heal yourself from microbial contamination and illness.

The Healing Properties of Coconut Oil

Coconut oil may help prevent illness or decrease its adverse effects once it strikes. In countries where coconut oil has been used for generations, it's considered an effective remedy for healing wounds. Some coconut-industry experts are working to have coconut oil officially classified as a nutraceutical, which is a dietary supplement or food that protects against or treats chronic diseases while contributing beneficial nutrients.

Coconut oil can actually boost the functioning of our immune systems, unlike unsaturated oils high in omega-6 fats, which can weaken the immune system by increasing inflammation and promoting cell growth. Coconut oil has even been shown to provide protection from six dangerous cancer-causing agents that interfere with DNA, including those found in cigarette smoke and diesel exhaust and possibly those in cooked meats cured with sodium nitrate.

Medium-Chain Fatty Acids in Coconut Oil

The following are the principal medium-chain fatty acids found in coconut oil:

- capric acid
- capryiic acid

- lauric acid
- myristic acid

How Coconut Oil Fights Microbes

Eighty percent of the medium-chain fatty acids in coconut oil have antimicrobial properties. Capric acid, caprylic acid, lauric acid, and myristic acid, all components of coconut oil, can interfere with the functioning of many harmful microorganisms. Of all of these, lauric acid, the principal fatty acid in coconut oil, has shown the greatest capability to defend against viruses and most bacteria.

Many bacteria and viruses are embodied in a capsule made up of fats. This coating protects microorganisms from drying up when they're outside of our bodies. The coating can also help an invading organism infect us, much like a burr would stick to a furry surface. By adhering to our skin, mucous membranes, and internal organs, the bacterium or virus can evade the body's immune defenses as if it had a bulletproof vest. Once inside us, bacteria and viruses use fats that are similar in structure to the medium-chain fatty acids in coconut oil to maintain this protective coating. If our diets include coconut oil, we'll have an increased chance that invading organisms will draw on these medium-chain fatty acids for their coatings rather than other fats. Unfortunately for the bacteria and viruses (but fortunately for us), medium-chain fatty acids don't maintain the integrity of this coating as well as other fatty acids do. This causes the membrane that protects invading organisms to disintegrate around them. The increased permeability of this membrane allows the entrance of molecules that bacteria and viruses would rather keep out; it also allows the release of molecules they would rather keep in.

People who have high concentrations of medium-chain fatty acids in their bodies have an extra line of defense protecting them from invading organisms. Our skin contains glands that continuously release protective oils that prevent the skin from drying out and becoming more susceptible to infection. The composition of this oil reflects the fats we consume; the more medium-chain fatty acids in our diets, the more medium-chain fats we'll have on our skin. A higher concentration of lauric acid on the skin can even help fight off the bacteria that cause pimples and acne. The medium-chain fatty acids that form coconut oil are the most potent at destroying bacteria and viruses. Of these, lauric acid is the most powerful, although all medium-chain fatty acids show some ability to destroy these organisms.

Coconut oil can be a great tool for defeating infectious bacteria. It's been shown to defend against the organisms that cause meningitis, several sexually transmitted diseases, staph infections, stomach upset, toxic shock syndrome, and ulcers; it also reduces dental caries up to 80 percent. Worldwide, there are approximately fifty million new cases every year of *Chlamydia trachomatis*, the most common sexually transmitted bacterial disease; this includes around four million cases in the United States alone. A study done in Iceland on the effectiveness of medium-chain fatty acids against chlamydia found that although high concentrations of capric acid were slightly more effective at reducing the numbers of all viable bacteria, lauric acid was much more effective, specifically against chlamydia, when both lauric and capric acids were used at a lower concentration.[20] The concentration of lauric acid used in this study more closely approximates the level you would obtain through the consumption of coconut oil.

Coconut Oil and Ulcers

Stress was once thought to be the main cause of ulcers. Although stress can be responsible for the onset of many illnesses, it now has been shown that the bacterium *Helicobacter pylori* is the principal cause of chronic gastritis and about 90 percent of peptic ulcers. Treatments with antibiotics have shown promise, but unfortunately the percentage of infections that return is very high, mostly due to people not taking their medications correctly. The side effects of the treatment are unpleasant, leading many people to misuse the drugs given to them. As a result, doctors are seeing more and more antibiotic resistance from *H. pylori* bacteria.

The greatest advantage to fighting organisms with medium-chain fatty acids is that bacteria and viruses don't commonly develop a resistance to them. The reasons for this are not yet clear to researchers, but one theory is that the effect of medium-chain fatty acids on the very structure of invading organisms is too great for the organisms' adaptive abilities to overcome.

Research has revealed another interesting key that correlates the success of coconut oil with the fact that it's saturated. When a mono-unsaturated form of lauric acid was tested alongside the saturated form, the saturated form was several thousand times more effective at destroying bacteria than its monounsaturated counterpart.[21] Also, lauric acid was the only fat shown to be effective at destroying *H. pylori*.

Lauric acid will still work against *H. pylori* even in the acidic conditions found in the stomach. Although stomach acid is strong enough to kill off many unwanted organisms, it isn't effective enough to destroy all infectious bacteria and viruses. In laboratory conditions, studies done with acid solutions containing *H. pylori* showed that the addition of glycerol monocaprate (monocaprin) and lauric acid effectively destroyed much of these bacteria. In fact, an acidic environment actually *increased* the potency of the mono-caprin and lauric acid to ward off *H. pylori*. Because of this, there should be a similar result in the acidic conditions of the stomach.

Coconut Oil and Yeast Infections

Not only could coconut oil decrease dependence on antibiotics, but it may also help to maintain a healthy balance of intestinal flora. One of the discouraging side effects of antibiotic treatment is that helpful bacteria are destroyed along with harmful bacteria. Certain friendly bacteria are actually needed to maintain health; for instance, these good bacteria aid with digestion and produce an acidic waste substance that reduces yeast levels in the body.

Candida albicans is a type of yeast that normally lives in small numbers around the oral cavity, lower gastrointestinal tract, and female genital tract. When the body's defenses are lowered, an overgrowth of yeast can cause many problems and discomforts.

The body's immune system works in concert with bacterial organisms that compete with the yeast for living space. Many infections caused by *C. albicans* occur when a dose of broad-spectrum antibiotics kills off helpful bacteria. In addition to coconut oil's potential for reducing the need for antibiotics, the fats in coconut oil may actually help destroy *Candida albicans* cells.

The same team of researchers that investigated the effect of capric acid and lauric acid on chlamydia also studied how fats affected three different strains of *C. albicans*. They found that capric acid and lauric acid were the only two fatty acids tested that had any substantial effect.[22] Just as it proved when fighting chlamydia, capric acid was most effective when the fatty acids were at a high concentration. However, lauric acid was most efficient when the concentration of fatty acids was lowered.

Coconut Oil and the Fight Against HIV and AIDS

HIV and its associated disease, AIDS, affect countless people around the world. Reducing the amount of HIV in the body has been a promising way to abate the onset of AIDS. An HIV-infected individual may live many healthy years before the disease progresses.

HIV mutates more than most viruses do because of the way it replicates. Each of the many variations of the virus may not be susceptible to the same drugs, and this increases the possibility of resistance to the drugs used against them. Consequently, a cocktail of drugs is typically used to combat the disease. The use of these drug combinations has been credited for a decline in AIDS deaths in many wealthy nations. Unfortunately, most of these drugs have undesirable side effects, including appetite suppression, nausea, muscle wasting, and displaced fat deposits that can lead to high cholesterol levels. Sadly, this increase in cholesterol can cause fatal heart attacks and lead to premature death before AIDS complications set in years later. These side effects have led numerous patients to seek out alternative treatments.

For many individuals, there are few treatment options. At present, many HIV-affected individuals live in developing nations, and a majority of those are in Africa. Drug cocktails are not readily available in less-developed countries, and when they are, they're very expensive, easily costing over $15,000 per person each year. These areas of the world would greatly benefit from an inexpensive treatment alternative.

Coconut oil not only has the potential to be an effective tool for fighting HIV, but it may also help ease the symptoms of AIDS and the troublesome side effects of the drugs used to treat this illness. In addition, both coconuts and coconut oil are more readily available than many medications and are much less expensive. HIV might be destroyed by coconut oil in much the same way as coconut oil destroys other susceptible bacteria and viruses.

Recently there's been much discussion and research on how a particular human herpes virus, HHV-6A, can work synergistically with HIV to promote the onset of AIDS. Fortunately, HHV-6A is one of the viruses killed by the medium-chain fatty acids found in coconut oil. HIV and HHV-6A incorporate medium-chain fatty acids into their protective coating, which then disintegrates around them. One study concluded the following: "This initial trial confirmed the anecdotal reports that coconut oil does have an antiviral effect and can beneficially reduce the viral load of HIV patients. The positive antiviral action was seen not only with the monoglyceride of lauric acid but with coconut oil itself. . . . With such products, the outlook for more efficacious and cheaper anti-HIV therapy is improved."[23] In the same study, eleven out of fifteen subjects gained weight, ranging from 4.5 to 50 pounds.

The recommended amount of coconut oil in a therapeutic dose is 3½ tablespoons per day. This equals the amount of oil found in approximately one-half of one coconut (about 1 cup grated), or 45 milliliters (22 grams) of monolaurin, which is formed from lauric acid. Monolaurin capsules can be helpful, but the same amount of monolaurin can be obtained by directly eating coconut oil, which contains other beneficial medium-chain fatty acids.

Coconut oil may deactivate many of the infections known to be a common complication for people who are HIV positive. It also may help the body maintain a healthy weight, a significant consideration for patients with HIV, AIDS, and other diseases that can cause wasting. Coconut oil could help undernourished individuals gain weight while not adding excess pounds to people with a weight problem.[24]

Coconut oil can also provide nutritional support during medical treatment. It's easily digested and known for providing energy more readily than other high-fat sources. Coconut oil has a very light flavor and a creamy texture, so it's convenient to incorporate into recipes, such as soups, smoothies, baked goods, oatmeal, and many other foods. It also may help improve overall immune system health and provide an extra defense against other opportunistic organisms.

Looking Toward the Future

Antibiotic use may be on the decline, especially for childhood illnesses. This offers some hope that we may be able to win the battle against antibiotic resistance. With the growing interest in alternative treatments for both chronic and acute illnesses, there certainly may be a place for coconut and coconut oil to be used with success. The nutritional stigma against coconut oil seems to be waning, and as a result, more research into its nutraceutical potential is sure to follow.

Coconut Oil for Beauty

It's no accident that people living in regions where coconut oil is used both in the diet and for body care have beautiful skin and hair. The healthy properties of coconut oil are not only effective internally but they also help promote a radiant glow all over.

Substances known as free radicals can influence both our internal and external health. Free radicals are unstable molecules that cause unwanted chemical reactions in the body. They can damage proteins, fats, cell membranes, and vital DNA, as well as contribute to the acceleration of the aging process. Because of their chemical structure, unsaturated oils are more prone to free radical damage. In their natural state, as part of whole nuts, seeds, and grains, they come packaged with protective antioxidants that limit free radical damage. When unsaturated oils are removed from their protective coverings, they become more susceptible to a chemical chain reaction that degrades their quality. Because coconut oil is a stable saturated fat, it's not broken down by free radicals. When it's used to replace unsaturated fats in our foods or applied to our skin, the opportunity for free radical damage is reduced and the aging process slows down.

The antimicrobial properties of coconut oil also extend to the skin and can help us look healthier and more beautiful. In addition, coconut oil has been shown to help combat acne and promote healing. Of course, using coconut oil in your cooking will feed your hair and skin from the inside out. A nutritious diet that includes high-quality, unrefined coconut oil can improve the appearance of hair and skin and give new meaning to the term "beauty from within."

Skin Care

Many people experience dry skin after being out in the sun any time of the year or during the winter months when the air inside and outside our homes is much less humid than in the summer. Dry skin also can be more of a problem as we age. Even people who have had very oily skin for much of their lives can experience dry skin in their later years on their legs and arms, where there are fewer oil glands than other areas of the body.

Coconut oil can be an effective natural alternative to expensive skin creams and lotions. Water-based lotions are so readily absorbed by the skin that they leave it feeling as dry as it was before they were applied. Many commercial lotions contain unwanted chemicals and unsaturated oils. Because a coconut is covered by several protective layers, even nonorganic coconut oils are relatively free of chemicals, pesticides, and herbicides. However, if you can't obtain organic coconut oil, be sure the product you buy is expeller pressed, not refined, so that it's free of chemical solvents.

Just a little coconut oil can go a long way. One of the best times to rehydrate your skin is right after a bath or shower. Don't dry your skin completely. Leave it slightly damp, and then apply a thin layer of coconut oil to your legs, arms, and any other problem areas. If you apply it to your face, don't forget your lips. After you start using coconut oil on a daily basis, you'll notice how water beads on your skin more than it had previously. This means that the coconut oil has formed a protective layer on your skin.

If you have trouble with dry skin on your feet, especially cracks around your heels, massage coconut oil into your clean feet before bedtime, then cover them with a pair of clean socks. You'll notice the difference in just a few nights. You can also repair damaged, dry hands the same way by using coconut oil and an old pair of cotton gloves. Finally, coconut oil is much safer for delicate tissues than petroleum-based products, making it an ideal choice as a natural vaginal lubricant. Because organic coconut oil is free of the chemicals typically used during oil processing, such as solvents, its extra cost is worth the investment.

Enhance some coconut oil with your favorite aromatherapy oil. Chamomile, lavender, and rose essential oils are soothing; peppermint and rosemary are invigorating. Use about 15 drops of essential oil to every cup of coconut oil. The exact amount of essential oil to use will depend on the strength of its fragrance and your preference. Add a few drops at a time to the coconut oil and rub the mixture on your skin to test it before adding more essential oil.

For ease of application, combine the coconut oil and aromatherapy oil in a clean squeeze bottle, such as the small, travel-sized containers sold in drugstores and supermarkets. Prepare a small amount of the mixture at a time to ensure that the oil essences remain fresh. During the colder months, put the bottle of coconut oil under hot running water if it becomes too thick to use. The warmth will thin out the oil and make it easier to use. If you like, cut open capsules of vitamin E and add the contents to your coconut oil mixture, using about 1 tablespoon per cup of oil. Vitamin E is an excellent antioxidant and skin healer. For a gentle, safe makeup remover, apply coconut oil with a cotton ball or washcloth.

Try this simple exfoliating body rub to moisturize as well as remove dead skin cells and rejuvenate your skin:

Exfoliating Coconut Body Rub

⅔ cup brown sugar

⅓ cup full-fat coconut milk, warmed

1 tablespoon coconut oil (optional; add if skin is very dry)

Put all the ingredients in a small bowl and mix well. Let cool. Massage into your skin for several minutes. Rinse well. For an invigorating foot rub, add 1 to 2 teaspoons of peppermint exact.

Massage Oil

Massaging with coconut oil is a wonderful way to incorporate this healthy, luxurious oil into your skin while gaining the benefits of relaxation and touch. Seek out a professional massage therapist or a partner or friend whose touch is soothing to you. If you're able to control the setting for your massage, pick a room that's warm and quiet. Soothing instrumental music will add to the relaxing experience. Although professional massage tables are great, a few thick blankets or several towels over an exercise mat on the floor can also provide a comfortable surface without too much give. Just 1 to 2 tablespoons of coconut oil are all you'll need for an effective massage.

Hair Care

Coconut oil is a common ingredient in commercial shampoos and hair conditioners. However, you can use the oil directly on your hair, too. Just apply the oil to your hair 30 to 60 minutes before you shampoo. Use 2 tablespoons to ½ cup of coconut oil, depending on the thickness and length of your hair. Begin by massaging the oil into your scalp and letting it drip down. Add more oil if necessary so you can stroke it down the length of your hair with both hands. If you have the time, wrap your hair in a towel or catch any drips by covering your scalp with a plastic shower cap. Alternatively, use a plastic shopping bag, tucking it behind your ears and gathering the ends at the nape of your neck. Let your hair soak up the oil for 20 to 60 minutes before washing it out. In the summer, you can wrap up your hair like this before you work in your garden or yard; the warmth of the sun will help your hair absorb more of the oil. It's hard to beat the feel of a soothing, cleansing shower after working outdoors and having a coconut oil hair treatment. Take extra precautions against slipping on the shower floor as you rinse out the oil.

Commercial Processes for Making Coconut Oil

The modern commercial method for making coconut oil and other foods from coconut usually involves drying the coconut meat and extracting the oil with solvents, the same as is done with the processing of most commercial vegetable oils. The oil is then deodorized to make a bland product that will more easily fit the needs of commercial food processors. This type of oil is often called RBD coconut oil, which stands for refined, bleached, and deodorized.

Omega Nutrition of Vancouver, Canada, and Bellingham, Washington, is an excellent source for organic coconut oil. The company recognized the importance of coconut oil in the early 1990s, a time when the oil was being vilified as a suspected contributor to heart disease. Omega Nutrition was the first company to reintroduce coconut oil to the natural food industry. Combined with the considerable efforts of biochemist and nutritionist Mary

Enig, Omega Nutrition paved the way for many other companies selling coconut oil today. Dr. Enig has worked tirelessly to provide consumers with the correct nutritional information for coconut oil and other tropical oils.

Omega Nutrition uses a special process to carefully remove the coconut flavor from their oil without using chemical solvents or damaging the oil's healthy properties. The result is a highly versatile product with a neutral flavor that can be used in any recipe. Coconut oils produced by many other manufacturers have a distinct coconut flavor, which may be wonderful in certain dishes but is not necessarily desirable in all.

Organic oil extraction processes also are springing up in various places around Southeast Asia. Tropical Traditions works with local coconut growers and processors in the Philippines, making a difference not only in the quality of its product but also in the quality of life in that country. By making its coconut oil with traditional processes that have been used for centuries, Tropical Traditions is able to pass on some of the financial benefits of its operation to small family businesses in the area.

Both Tropical Traditions and Garden of Life, another company that manufactures a popular brand of coconut oil, extract their oil by grating fresh coconut and either pressing the coconut milk from the fresh kernel or lightly drying the kernel and then pressing it. The extracted coconut milk is then fermented for twenty-four to thirty-six hours, at which point the oil rises to the top and separates out from the milk. Next, the oil is heated slightly to evaporate most of the remaining moisture; after that, it is filtered to remove any particles that remained from the pressing process. The result is an oil with rich coconut flavor and aroma.

Other organic coconut oil processing operations in Southeast Asia include those set up by the Women in Business Foundation on the island of Samoa, where rural village women employ traditional methods to make organic coconut oil. In the Caribbean, a brand of oil called Jamaican Gold is manufactured in small batches for Essential Oil Company by cold-pressing organic coconut meat that has been gently dehydrated.

Another commercial process used to make quality coconut oil involves centrifuging coconut milk made from grated fresh coconut. This separates the oil in the milk from the water and solids; the process uses no heat. Popular brands using this method are Coconut Oil Supreme and organic Nature's Blessings. There are also other top-quality brands of organic coconut oil appearing in the marketplace, such as Nutiva; these products are manufactured using a variety of processing methods. The growth of this industry attests to the increasing interest in using coconut oil for its health benefits.

Recipes

Coconut Fruit Salad

Makes 7 cups

This tasty fruit salad is quick and easy, and the kiwifruit and mandarin oranges add a delightful twist. Use larger coconut flakes if you can find them; they'll add great flavor along with eye appeal.

1 fresh pineapple, cut into chunks (about 4 cups)

2 (11-ounce) cans mandarin orange sections packed in juice, drained

2 kiwifruit, peeled, halved, and sliced

⅓ cup unsweetened shredded dried coconut

1 tablespoon freshly squeezed lemon juice

1 cup freshly squeezed orange juice

Put the pineapple, orange sections, kiwifruit, and coconut in a large bowl. Stir the lemon juice into the orange juice and pour over the fruit mixture. Stir to combine. Cover and refrigerate until thoroughly chilled.

Tofu Vegetable Curry

Makes 4 servings

This recipe showcases the Indian culinary practice of tempering spices in oil. Serve this curry over cooked brown rice or quinoa.

2 tablespoons coconut oil

1 teaspoon whole cumin seeds

1 teaspoon ground turmeric

1 teaspoon ground coriander

½ teaspoon salt

1 pound extra-firm tofu, cut into ½-inch cubes

2 carrots, scrubbed and sliced

1 cup frozen peas

1 cup full-fat coconut milk

¼ cup water or vegetable broth

½ teaspoon crushed red pepper flakes (optional)

Heat the coconut oil in a large, heavy skillet over medium heat. Add the cumin seeds and fry just until the seeds just begin to sizzle and brown, 1 to 2 minutes. Add the turmeric, coriander, and salt and cook, stirring frequently, for 1 minute. Add the tofu, carrots, and peas and stir to combine. Cook, stirring frequently, until the carrots start to soften, 5 to 10 minutes. Add the coconut milk, water, and optional pepper flakes. Cover and cook over low heat, stirring occasionally, until the vegetables are tender, about 20 minutes. Serve hot.

Pacific Rim Rice

Makes 4 servings

This tropical pilaf is rich and satisfying, and the cashews contribute a delicious crunch.

3 tablespoons coconut oil
1 onion, finely chopped
1 green bell pepper, finely chopped
¾ teaspoon curry powder
3 cups vegetable stock, hot
1½ cups brown basmati rice
¾ cup full-fat coconut milk
¼ teaspoon salt
1 cup pineapple chunks
¼ cup chopped unsalted roasted or raw cashews

Heat the coconut oil in a medium saucepan over medium heat. Add the onion and bell pepper and cook, stirring frequently, until the onion is golden brown, about 10 minutes. Stir in the curry powder and cook, stirring frequently, for 1 minute. Remove from the heat and slowly stir in the hot vegetable stock. Bring to a simmer over high heat. Stir in the rice, coconut milk, and salt. Decrease the heat to medium, cover, and simmer until no liquid is visible at the bottom of the pan when you tilt it, about 30 minutes. Remove from the heat and stir in the pineapple and cashews. Cover and let sit for 10 minutes before serving to let all the remaining moisture be absorbed.

Mashed Sweet Potatoes with Coconut

Makes 4 servings

This easy recipe has uncommonly good flavor and is one of our favorites.

4 medium sweet potatoes, peeled and quartered

2 tablespoons coconut oil

1 onion, chopped

½ cup orange juice

¼ cup unsweetened shredded dried coconut

Salt

Put the sweet potatoes in a medium saucepan and cover with water. Bring to a boil over high heat. Decrease the heat to medium-high and simmer until soft, 10 to 15 minutes. Drain well. Transfer to a large bowl and mash.

While the sweet potatoes are cooking, heat the oil in a medium skillet over medium-high heat. Add the onion and cook, stirring frequently, until tender and starting to brown, about 10 minutes.

Add the onion, orange juice, and coconut to the sweet potatoes and stir to combine. Season with salt to taste.

Yellow Split Pea and Coconut Soup

Makes 4 servings

Dishes in southern India frequently include coconut in a variety of forms. Enjoy this soup on its own or serve it as an Indian sambar or kootu over basmati rice.

1 cup dried yellow split peas

4 cups water

¼ cup coconut oil

1 teaspoon ground turmeric

½ teaspoon whole cumin seeds

½ teaspoon ground ginger

1 onion, chopped

1 tablespoon minced garlic

½ cup unsweetened shredded dried coconut

Put the split peas in a large soup pot. Add the water and bring to a boil over medium-high heat. Decrease the heat to medium and simmer, stirring frequently, until the split peas are soft and breaking apart, about 45 minutes.

Heat the coconut oil in a medium skillet over medium-high heat. Add the turmeric, cumin seeds, and ginger and cook, stirring almost constantly, until the seeds just begin to sizzle and brown, 1 to 2 minutes. Decrease the heat to low, add the onion and garlic, and cook, stirring frequently, until the onion is golden, 5 to 10 minutes. Add the coconut and stir to combine. Stir the coconut mixture into the split peas. Reheat over medium heat, stirring frequently, until hot.

Nutritional Properties of Coconut

Fresh coconut (1.6 ounces; one 2 x 2-inch piece, ½-inch thick)

calories	177
protein	1.7 grams
fat	16.8 grams
saturated fat	14.8 grams
carbohydrates	7.6 grams
fiber	4.5 grams
potassium	178 grams
phosphorus	57 milligrams
magnesium	16 milligrams

Dried coconut (¾ cup)

calories	334
protein	3.6 grams
fat	32.7 grams
saturated fat	29 grams
carbohydrates	12 grams
fiber	17 grams
potassium	275 grams
phosphorus	100 milligrams
magnesium	46 milligrams

GLOSSARY

Antioxidants. Substances that inhibit oxidation and help prevent the degradation of organic compounds and the formation of free radicals are called antioxidants.

Cholesterol. The waxy substance known as cholesterol is created in our bodies from small molecules of acetate that result primarily from the breakdown of fats and sugars and in some circumstances protein.

Fatty acids. The building blocks of fats are fatty acids, which are chains of carbon and hydrogen atoms, each with a group of oxygen and hydrogen atoms at the end.

Free radicals. Unstable molecules called free radicals scavenge throughout the body for stable molecules they can raid for oxygen atoms.

High-density lipoprotein. More commonly referred to as HDL, high-density lipoprotein is a lipoprotein that removes cholesterol from the blood and is associated with a reduced risk of atherosclerosis and heart disease.

Hydrogenation. The process used to transform liquid oils into artificially solid fats is called hydrogenation. During this process, hydrogen atoms are added to the double bonds of unsaturated carbon chains, creating a straightened chain without any unstable bonds.

Low-density lipoprotein. More commonly referred to as LDL, low-density lipoprotein is a lipoprotein that transports cholesterol in the blood. It is composed of a moderate amount of protein and a large amount of cholesterol. High levels are thought to be associated with increased risk of coronary heart disease and atherosclerosis.

Nutraceutical. A dietary supplement or food that protects against or treats chronic diseases while also contributing to better nutrition is known as a nutraceutical.

Omega-3 fatty acid. An essential fatty acid, omega-3 is a polyunsaturated fatty acid that must be obtained through diet because the body cannot synthesize it. Omega-3 fatty acid can help lower blood pressure and reduce inflammation.

Omega-6 fatty acid. Omega-6 fatty acid is a polyunsaturated fatty acid found in oils. Excessive consumption of omega-6 fatty acids is believed to raise blood pressure, increase inflammation, and lead to certain diseases.

RBD coconut oil. Coconut oil that has been refined, bleached, and deodorized is referred to as RBD.

Trans fats. Trans fats are manufactured from polyunsaturated fats and have properties that more closely resemble saturated fats.

REFERENCES

1. Ascherio, A., et al. "Dietary fat and risk of coronary heart disease in men," *BMJ* (1996): 313:84–90.

2. Sundram, K., et al. "Replacement of dietary fat with palm oil: effect on human serum lipids, lipoproteins and apoliproteins," *British Journal of Nutrition* (November 1992): 68(3):677–92.

3. de Roos, Nicole M., et al. "Consumption of a solid fat rich in lauric acid results in a more favorable serum lipid profile in healthy men and women than consumption of a solid fat rich in trans-fatty acids," *Journal of Nutrition* (2001): 131:242–245.

4. Sadeghi, S., et al. "Dietary lipids modify the cytokine response to bacterial lipopolysaccharide in mice," *Immunology* (March 1999): 96(3):404–10.

5. Nelson, S. E., et al. "Palm olein in infant formula: absorption of fat and minerals by normal infants," *American Journal of Clinical Nutrition* (1996): 64:291–296.

6. Cohen, L. A. "Medium chain triglycerides lack tumor-promoting effects in the n-methylnitrosourea-induced mammary tumor model," *The Pharmacological Effects of Lipids*, edited by Jon J. Kabara. (1998): 3. The American Oil Chemists' Society.

7. Kabara, Jon J. "Nutritional and health aspects of coconut oil," *Indian Coconut Journal* (2000): 31(8):2–8.

8. St-Onge, Marie-Pierre, P. J. H. Jones. "Physiological effects of medium-chain triglycerides: potential agents in the prevention of obesity," *Journal of Nutrition* (2002): 132:/3/29–332.

9. Portillo, M. P., et al. "Energy restriction with high-fat diet enriched with coconut oil gives higher UCP1 and lower white fat in rats," *International Journal of Obesity and Related Metabolic Disorders* (1998): 22:974–9.

10. Kaunitz, Hanz and C. S. Dayrit. "Coconut oil consumption and coronary heart disease," *Philippine Journal of Internal Medicine* (1992): 30:165–171.

11. Kumar, P. D. "The role of coconut and coconut oil in coronary heart disease in Kerala, South India," *Tropical Doctor.* (October 1997): 27(4):215–217.

12. Ng, T. K. W., et al. "Nonhypercholesterolemic effects of a palm-oil diet in Malaysian volunteers," *American Journal of Clinical Nutrition* (1991): 53:1015S–1020S.

13. Sundaram, K., et al. "Dietary palmitic acid results in lower serum cholesterol than does a lauric myristic combination in normolipemic humans," *American Journal of Clinical Nutrition* (1994): 59:371–377.

14. Thampan, P. K. *Facts and Fallacies about Coconut Oil,* Jakarta: Asian and Pacific Coconut Community, 1998.

15. Mendis, S., et al. "The effects of replacing coconut oil with corn oil on human serum lipid profiles and platelet derived factors active in atherogenesis," *Nutrition Reports International* (October 1989): 40:No.4.

16. Prior, I. A., et al. "Cholesterol, coconuts, and diet on Polynesian atolls: a natural experiment: the Pukapuka and Tokelau Island studies," *American Journal of Clinical Nutrition* (1981): 34:1552–1561.

17. See note 14.

18. Satcher, David. "Emerging infections: getting ahead of the curve," *Emerging Infectious Diseases* (1995): 1(1):1–6.

19. Hughes, James M. "Emerging infectious diseases: A CDC perspective," *Emerging Infectious Diseases* (2001): 7(3):494–496.

20. Bergsson, Gudmundur, et al. "In vitro inactivation of chlamydia trachomatis by fatty acids and monoglycerides," *Antimicrobial Agents and Chemotherapy* (September 1998): 2290–2294.

21. Petschow, Byron W., et al. "Susceptibility of helicobacter pylori to bactericidal properties of medium-chain monglycerides and free fatty acids," *Antimicrobial Agents and Chemotherapy* (February 1996): 302–306.

22. Bergsson, Gudmundur, et al. "In vitro killing of candida albicans by fatty acids and monoglycerides," *Antimicrobial Agents and Chemotherapy* (November 2001): 3209–3212.

23. Dayrit, Conrad. "Coconut oil in health and disease: ITS and mono-laurin's potential as cure for HIV/AIDS." Paper presented at the XXXVII Cocotech Meeting, Chennai, India, July 25, 2000.

24. See note 23.

BIBLIOGRAPHY

Davis, Brenda, and Vesanto Melina. *Becoming Vegan: Comprehensive Edition*. Summertown, TN: Book Publishing Co., 2014.

Dinsdale, Margaret. *Skin Deep*. Buffalo, NY: Firefly Books, 1998.

Enig, Mary. *Know Your Fats*. Silver Spring, MD: Bethesda Press, 2000.

Erasmus, Udo. *Fats and Oils*. Vancouver: Books Alive, 2010.

Fife, Bruce. *The Coconut Oil Miracle*. New York: Avery/Penguin, 2013.

Gursche, Siegfried. *Good Fats and Oils*. Vancouver: Alive Books, 2000.

Lombard, Kevin. "Reviewing the Coconut (Cocos nucifera L.)." A paper written and presented for PSS 5326 Advanced Seed Science, Texas Tech University, 2001.

Regional Energy Resources Information Center (RERIC). "Desiccated Coconut Sector." Klong Luang, Thailand: Asian Institute of Technology, 2002.

Soyatech, Inc. *2014 Soya & Oilseed Bluebook*. Southwest Harbor, ME: Soyatech, Inc., 2013.

Woodroof, J.G. *Coconuts: Production, Processing, Products*. 2nd ed. Westport, CT: AVI Publishing Company, Inc., 1979.

Cookbooks with Coconut Recipes

Asian Fusion, Chat Mingkwan

Coconut Cuisine, Jan London

Raw for Dessert, Jennifer Cornbleet

Sweet Utopia, Sharon Valencik

ABOUT THE AUTHORS

Cynthia Holzapfel is a health editor and research writer specializing in vegetarian cooking and nutrition. As managing editor for Book Publishing Company, she has contributed to more than 100 cookbooks and health titles.

Laura Holzapfel is a health administrator and writer/researcher on women's health topics and vegetarian nutrition.

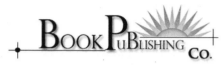

Book Publishing Co.

books that educate, inspire, and empower

A Holistic Approach to **ADHD** – *Deborah Merlin*

Weight Loss and Good Health with **APPLE CIDER VINEGAR** – *Cynthia Holzapfel*

The Weekend **DETOX** – *Jerry Lee Hutchens*

Improve Digestion with **FOOD COMBINING** – *Steve Meyerowitz*

Understanding **GOUT** – *Warren Jefferson*

PALEO Smoothies – *Alan Roettinger*

Refreshing Fruit and Vegetable **SMOOTHIES** – *Robert Oser*

All titles in the **Live Healthy Now** series are only **$5.95!**

Interested in other health topics or healthy cookbooks?
See our complete line of titles at bookpubco.com
or order directly from:

Book Publishing Company
P.O. Box 99
Summertown, TN 38483
1-888-260-8458